SOMATIC EXERCISE

For Women Over 40

Gentle exercise to enhance mobility, reduce pain, and boost wellbeing for women beyond 40

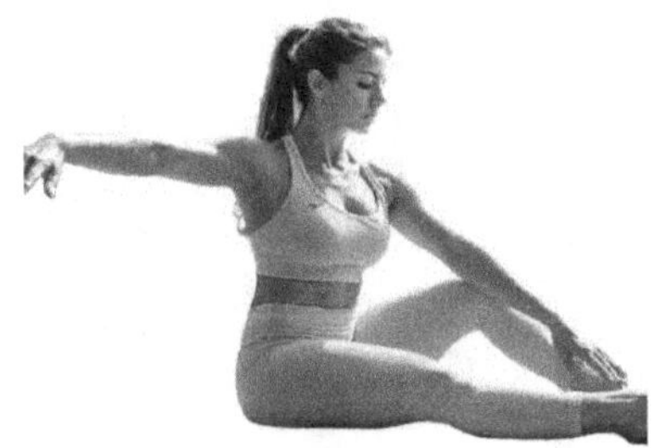

Matthew Brewer

DISCLAIMER

Table of Contents

Introduction

Do you ever feel separated from your body? As if it were a vehicle, you inhabited rather than a companion on your journey through life. For many women, the stresses of everyday life, cultural expectations, and even prior experiences can cause a disconnect between our brains and bodies. This connection can appear in a variety of ways, including chronic tension, aches and pains, a sense of discomfort, or a persistent sensation that something isn't quite right.

This is where somatic movement comes in, providing a powerful and transforming way to reclaim your body and mind. As someone who has spent years researching the realm of somatic exercise, I can assure you that it is more than just stretching and working out. Somatic movement is a voyage of rediscovery, a method to reconnect with your inner knowledge and realize your body's enormous potential.

Imagine moving with purpose, feeling the earth beneath your feet, and experiencing a delicate symphony of feelings within you. Somatic movement enables you to nurture this acute awareness, resulting in a better knowledge of how your body moves, feels, and responds to the world around you. It's about moving with tenderness, inquiry, and respect while acknowledging your own needs and limitations.

But why is somatic movement so vital for women, specifically? Throughout our lifetimes, we face a complicated environment of physical, mental, and hormonal changes. Somatic movement offers a safe environment to examine these changes while also providing tools for stress management, pain relief, and resilience development. It encourages you to take an active role in your own well-being, developing a sense of self-acceptance and confidence.

This book invites you to go on a transforming journey. Within these pages, you will learn about the tremendous advantages of somatic movement, moderate exercises for various body regions, and how to incorporate this practice into your daily life. Whether you're an experienced athlete or haven't exercised in years, somatic movement offers something for you. It's a practice that adapts to you, providing support and advice as you negotiate life's ever-changing environment. So, take a deep breath, walk onto the mat (or simply stand tall), and be ready to reconnect with the immense power that exists inside you.

Chapter 1: The Power of Present Moment Awareness.

Techniques for grounding and centering

Let's go to the voyage of embodied inquiry! Before we get started with somatic movement, let's lay the groundwork for present-moment awareness. This helps us to reconnect with our body, reduce mental chatter, and prepare for a more focused movement experience. Here are some grounding and centering methods intended exclusively for ladies and novices.

1. 5-4-3-2-1 Technique:

This easy technique focuses your attention on your immediate surroundings, anchoring you in the present moment. Find a comfortable and a quiet place and take a few deep breaths. Recognize five items you see around you (a picture, a plant, the color of the walls). Then, list four things you can feel (the texture of your clothes, the coldness of the floor under you). Next, concentrate on three sounds you can hear (traffic outside, refrigerator hum). Notice two things you can smell. Finally, focus on one taste. Repeat the exercise as many times as necessary to feel anchored.

2. Deep breathing for grounding:

Our breath is a very effective tool for connecting with our bodies and soothing our nervous systems. Find a comfortable sitting or standing position. Place one hand on your stomach, the other on your chest. Close your eyes gently (if comfortable) and inhale slowly and deeply through your nose. Feel your stomach expand as your lungs fill with air. Hold for a second before gently exhaling through pursed lips, feeling your tummy compress as you expel the breath. Repeat this breathing pattern for many minutes, concentrating on the rise and fall of your breath.

3. Body Scan:

This technique encourages you to softly scan your body from head to toe, becoming aware of any feelings that arise. Begin by resting comfortably on your back or sitting in a comfortable position. Shut your eyes and take multiple deep breaths. Mentally scan your body, starting with your toes. Take note of any sensations of tension, warmth, coldness, tingling, or a neutral sense. Continue to look upwards, recognizing each portion of your body without judgment. If your mind wanders, carefully return your attention to the body scan. Repeat the process as many times as you like.

4. Sensorial Walk:

This grounding approach helps you to connect with your surroundings using your senses. Take a stroll outside or just around your house. As you walk, take note of the sights, sounds, scents, textures, and even tastes (if safe) that surround you. Take note of the details: the way the sunshine filters through the leaves, the sound of birds tweeting, and the freshness of the grass beneath your bare feet (if comfortable). Immersion in the sensory environment naturally leads to a sense of presence and roundedness.

Remember, these are only a few beginning points. Experiment with several ways to see what resonates with you the best. The secret is to be patient and gentle to oneself. As you practice these exercises on a daily basis, you will develop a stronger connection to your body as well as a sense of serenity that you can carry with you throughout the day.

The importance of Breathwork in Somatic Movement

As we begin on this journey to reconnect with our bodies, we will always have one crucial instrument with us: our breath. Breathwork is more than just oxygenating your body; it is the link between your thoughts and your bodily feelings. Understanding and incorporating mindful breathing into your somatic practice will allow you to achieve a higher degree of awareness and maximize the potential of your movements.

Why Breath Matters in Somatic Movement

Improves Body Awareness: Focusing on your breath directs your focus within. You'll notice how your breath reacts to movement, where you retain stress, and how different parts of your body expand and compress.

Calms the Nervous System: Deep, calm breaths trigger your body's parasympathetic nervous system, or "rest and digest" response. This counteracts the fight-or-flight reaction, allowing you to move more freely and relieve stored stress.

Improves Movement Fluidity: Smooth and linked breathing allows for more fluid and coordinated motions. You'll discover a natural rhythm in your somatic practice, allowing for deeper investigation.
Simple techniques for beginners:

Now, let us put this information into practice! Here are two basic breathing methods to incorporate into your somatic movement journey:

1. Diaphragmatic Breath:
This is the normal method to breathe, using your diaphragm, a dome-shaped muscle beneath your lungs. This is how you do it:
- Lie comfortably on your back, one hand on your stomach and the other on your chest.
- As you softly inhale through your nose, let your belly gently push your hand outward. Your chest should be reasonably motionless.
- Exhale gently through pursed lips, allowing your belly to sink inwards as your hand follows.

2. Nostril breathing (alternate nostril breathing):

This approach helps to calm the mind and induce relaxation. Here's how to practice it:

- Sit comfortably with a straight spine.
- Gently seal your right nostril with your thumb.
- Inhale gently via the left nostril.
- Hold your breath for a comfortable count (optional).
- Close your left nostril with your ring finger, then gently exhale through your right nose.
- Inhale via your right nostril, hold (optional), then expel through your left nostril.
- Repeat this pattern for a few breaths, switching sides.

Integrating Breathwork with Somatic Movement:

As you experiment with different somatic exercises, utilize your breath to direct your motions. Here are a few tips:

- Synchronize your breath with your movement: inhale as you begin an opening movement (for example, stretching your arms aloft), and exhale as you return to neutral.
- Concentrate on the exhale: Use the exhalation to relieve tension and facilitate deeper stretches.
- Listen to your body: If you experience any discomfort, modify your breathing or the action itself.

Remember that breathwork is a journey, not a destination. Be patient with yourself, and as you practice consistently, you'll notice that your breath becomes a natural extension of your somatic movement, allowing you to move with more awareness, ease, and grace.

Chapter 2: Exploring Your Body Landscape.

Body Scans: Tuning Into Internal Sensations

Welcome to the realm of somatic movements! Our trip starts with a fundamental practice: the body scan. This simple yet effective approach helps us develop present-moment awareness and become intimately familiar with our interior sensations.

Imagine your body as a place to be explored. A body scan transforms us into interested explorers, carefully roaming our inner environment and noting small nuances. This technique does not include passing judgment or pressing change, but rather watching with love and acceptance.

<u>**Here's how you can do a body scan:**</u>
Find a Quiet Space:
Choose a peaceful, comfortable environment where you will not be bothered. Lie down on a mat or sit erect in a chair, feet flat on the floor.
Grounding yourself:

Take a few deep breaths, gently inhaling with your nose and fully expelling through your mouth. Feel your body sink into the surface underneath you.
Beginning the scan:

Close your eyes lightly, or lower your gaze if you like. Bring your attention to your toes. Feel any feelings there - warmth, coldness, tingling, or a sense of pressure on the mat. Simply observe rather than analyzing.

Slowly shift your focus upward, experiencing the feelings in each region of your body - your feet, ankles, calves, and so on. Pay close attention to any tension, tightness, or relaxation.

Continue to inspect your legs, chest, arms, hands, neck, and head.

As you scan, you may discover places of tension. Recognize them without judgment. If it helps, picture sending a soft wave of breath to those places, encouraging relaxation.

<u>Ending the Scan:</u>
After you've inspected your entire body, take a few deep breaths. Gently twitch your fingers and toes before gently opening your eyes (if closed).

<u>Bringing Awareness to Daily Life:</u>
The beauty of body scans is that they can be performed anywhere at any time. Throughout the day, pause to check in with your body. Consider your posture, any places of tension, or just the sensation of your breath going in and out.

<u>Tips for Beginners:</u>
- Do not worry if your thoughts stray throughout the scan. Gently return your full attention to your body.
- Body scans can be both brief and lengthy. Begin with a few minutes and progressively increase the time as you feel more comfortable.
- If any sensations make you uncomfortable, move your attention to another location or stop the scan.

- The more you perform body scans, the more aware you will become of your body's subtle messages.

By practicing present-moment awareness via body scans, you'll go on a transforming journey of self-discovery and lay the groundwork for a more embodied and empowered existence.

Sensory Awareness Exercises for Sight, Sound, Touch, Smell, and Taste

---

Let's dip in wonderful world within! Before we go into particular somatic exercises, let's wake up our senses and develop a stronger connection to our interior world. This increased awareness will lay the groundwork for your somatic practice.

Sensory awareness activities encourage you to be an inquisitive observer of your own experience. We'll investigate each of the five senses - sight, hearing, touch, smell, and taste - via simple, common activities.

<u>Find a Quiet Space:</u>
Set out a few minutes in a quiet, comfortable environment to fully engage in these activities. Turn off any distractions, be it phones or televisions.
The Art of Observation:

Approach each exercise with calm inquiry. Do not criticize or analyze your experience; instead, simply observe.

<u>Ready? Let us begin!</u>

1. Seeing
Observe the ordinary: Sit comfortably and look about the room. Examine the colors, textures, and forms of items. Is there a dance of light and shadow that you hadn't seen before? Take a time to admire the beauty of the mundane.

2) Hearing:
The Symphony of noises: Close your eyes and concentrate on the noises surrounding you. Can you discriminate between close and remote sounds? Are there varying pitches or rhythms? Perhaps you hear the hum of a refrigerator or the buzz of birds. Appreciate your surroundings' distinct soundscape.

3. Touch.

Feel Your Breath: Place one hand on your chest and the other on your abdomen. Observe the delicate rise and fall with each breath. Is your breathing shallow or deep?

How do the temperatures in your hands differ? Be conscious of the bodily feelings of breathing.

Exploring Textures: Gently close your eyes and grasp a familiar object, such as a piece of fruit or a silky scarf. Examine the texture against your skin. Is it smooth, rough, cool, or warm? Explore diverse textures throughout the day, such as the softness of your garments and the coldness of a bottle of water.

4. Smell

Aromatic Awareness: Light a fragrant candle (if you have one) or open a container with a pleasant odor, such as coffee beans or essential oils. Take a deep breath and breath in the fragrance. Where can you smell it the most strongly? Does it bring up any memories or emotions?

5. Taste.

Savoring the Simple: Take a taste of fruit or a basic cracker. Chew gently, observing the texture and flavor. Can you identify diverse taste sensations such as sweet, sour, salty, and bitter? Pay attention to how the flavors vary while you chew.

Beyond the exercises:

Integrating these sensory awareness exercises into your everyday routine is critical. Take a careful bite of your food, fully listen to the sounds of nature while walking, or admire the delicate intricacies of a flower. By increasing your sensory awareness, you will get a better knowledge of your body and its relationship to the world around you.

Remember:

There are no correct or incorrect responses in these activities. Accept the road of discovery and cherish the unique way you see the world via your senses. This heightened awareness will be a valuable asset in your somatic movement practice.

Chapter 3: Find Freedom in Your Spine: Gentle Mobility Exercises

Exercises for Neck and Shoulder Release

Tightness in the neck and shoulders is a frequent symptom, typically caused by stress, poor posture, or overuse. The good news is that a few simple somatic motions can provide relief and relaxation.

Here are three beginner-friendly exercises you can do anywhere, anytime to relieve stress in your neck and shoulders.

1. Ear-to-shoulder stretch:

- **Starting position:** Sit or stand tall, shoulders relaxed and down.
- Gently tilt your head to one side, bringing your ear near your shoulder. You should feel a bit stretch on the side of your neck.
- **Hold and Breathe:** Maintain this posture for 15-30 seconds while breathing deeply and slowly. Concentrate on the sensation of the stretch without straining it.
- Repeat and switch sides. Gently return your head to the center and repeat the stretch on the opposite side. Aim for 2-3 reps per side.

2) Neck Rolls:

- **Starting position:** Sit or stand tall, shoulders relaxed and down.
- **Gentle Movement:** Begin slowly turning your head in a circular motion, as if saying "no" with your chin. To achieve a softer movement, lead with your chin rather than your neck.
- **Breathe and Flow:** Make many rounds in one direction, concentrating on your breath and any points of tension. Then, reverse the direction and do many more circles.

3. <u>Doorway Chest Opener (Shoulder Release):</u>

- **Finding Your Anchor:** Stand in a doorway, arms beside the doorframe. Bend your elbows at 90 degrees and place your forearms flat against the doorframe on either side, around shoulder height.
- **tilt In and Breathe:** Slowly tilt your chest forward, allowing a mild stretch over your chest and shoulders. Maintain a modest bend in your knees to avoid overextending them. Breathe deeply and hold for 15-30 seconds.
- **Release and Repeat:** Gently return to the beginning position and repeat the stretch 2-3 times.

<u>Tips for Beginners:</u>

Listen to Your Body: These movements should feel like a mild stretch and produce no discomfort. If you are uncomfortable, slow down or stop the exercise.

Focus on Breath: Throughout these stretches, concentrate on your breathing. Inhale slowly and deeply, then exhale fully with each release.

Small motions, Big Impact: Do not push huge motions. For best benefits, focus on tiny, soft stretches that may be held for an extended amount of time.

Make it a Habit: Perform these exercises throughout the day, especially if you have stress in your neck and shoulders.

By implementing these basic stretches into your daily routine, you may relieve tension, improve your posture, and encourage relaxation in your neck and shoulders.

Spinal Articulation and Lengthening Sequence

The spine is our body's core, sustaining our posture and providing a wide range of motion. However, regular activity and stress can cause stiffness and strain in the spine. This chapter covers moderate articulation and lengthening sequences for improving mobility and creating a sensation of relaxation in your back.

<u>Important Reminders:</u>

- **Listen to Your Body:** Prioritize comfort above flawless posture. Modify the exercises as appropriate, and stop if you feel pain.
- **Slow and steady wins the race.** Concentrate on smooth, controlled motions. Allow your breath to drive your movements: inhale as you expand, and exhale as you release.

<u>**Gentle Spinal Articulation:**</u>

1. Cat-Cow: Start on all fours, hands shoulder-width apart and both knees hip-width apart. * Inhale, arch your back slightly and raise your head and tailbone (cow position). Feel your spine stretch and your chest expand. Exhale, round your back, and bury your chin into your chest (cat stance). Feel your spine bend inwards and your core engage. Repeat this mild wave-like motion 5-10 times while matching your breath with the action.

2. Spinal Twists (Seated or Standing): Sit on the floor or stand with feet hip-width apart.
Inhale and stretch one arm above to lengthen your spine. Exhale and slowly twist your torso to the side, stretching your opposing arm behind you to stretch your side and chest. Maintain a forward-facing hip position and avoid twisting the neck. Hold for a few breaths before inhaling and returning to center. Repeat on the opposite side.

<u>**Extending Sequences:**</u>

1. Children's Pose with Arm Reaches: Kneel on the floor, toes together, knees hip-width apart. Sit back on your heels, resting your forehead on the mat.
Stretch your both arms out in front of you, palms facing downward. Experience a nice stretch in your lower back and shoulders. Hold for 5-10 breaths before gently walking your hands back towards your hips to return to a sitting posture.

2. Supine Spinal Waves: Lie on your back, legs bent, feet flat on the floor. Place your arms at your sides. * Gently press your lower back into the mat while taking a deep breath and raising your head and shoulders off the floor. Hold for a second before slowly exhaling and lowering yourself back down. * Repeat this wave-like action 5-10 times, focusing on starting the movement with your spine rather than your neck.

Remember:

These are only a starting point! As you grow more familiar with these exercises, try other variants that target different parts of your spine. You may try neck rolls, moderate side bends, or resting on your back with your legs bent and swaying side to side.

The objective is to move with intention and awareness, creating a sensation of comfort and movement in your spine. With persistent practice, you'll experience increased mobility and lightness in your back.

Techniques to Improve Posture

Beautiful posture is more than simply looking beautiful; it also feels good! Proper alignment may increase your energy, relieve discomfort, and promote your confidence. What is the best part? You may start practicing proper posture right now with a few basic strategies.

Here's a step-by-step strategy for improving your posture.

Stand tall.

- Consider a cord tugging you upward from the crown of your head. This simple stretch lengthens your spine and helps with general alignment.
- Relax your shoulders and let them slide down your back. Avoid hunching them forwards.
- Engage your core muscles. Imagine softly moving your belly button toward your spine. This offers stability and support for your back.
- Keep your feet hip-width apart and spread your weight equally. Place your knees slightly bent rather than locking them.

<u>**Sitting Tall:**</u>

- Choose a chair that provides decent back support. The backrest should bend slightly to support your lower back.
- Sit all the way back in your chair and adjust the seat height so that your knees are bent at a 90° angle. Your feet should be flat on the floor.
- Maintain the spinal alignment you used when standing. Extend your spine, prevent slouching, and maintain your shoulders relaxed.
- If your chair lacks enough lumbar support, consider utilizing a rolled-up towel or lumbar cushion to provide additional support in your lower back.

<u>**Mindfulness During the Day:**</u>

- Set reminders. Set mild reminders throughout the day (for example, an alarm on your phone) to check your posture. Are you slouching? Gently alter your position.
- Engage in activities that encourage proper posture. Yoga, Pilates, and even brief periods of standing against a wall can help strengthen the muscles that promote healthy posture.

- Start slowly and be patient. Building proper posture requires time and constant work. Celebrate even minor improvements!
- Listen to your body. If you encounter any pain, stop exercising and get medical attention.
- Concentrate on feeling good, not looking flawless. Good posture should be natural and pleasant, not stiff or forced.

Remember, consistency is crucial! By implementing these strategies into your everyday routine, you'll be well on your way to mastering your posture and feeling your best.

Exercise Positions for Various Body Sections

Spine

Cat-Cow Pose

The cat-cow stance is an essential movement in both yoga and somatic exercises. It gently stretches and mobilizes your spine, increasing flexibility and posture.

Here's a step-by-step instruction to help novices do the cat-cow stance with ease:

Starting Position (table pose):
1. Begin on your hands and knees, with your hands shoulder-width apart and squarely beneath your shoulders.
2. Knees should be hip width apart, toes tucked under or flat on the floor.
3. Maintain a neutral spine by aligning your head with your spine and gazing down slightly in front of you.
4. Take a few deep breaths to help you relax and feel at ease in this posture.

Moving to Cow Pose (Exhale):
1. As you exhale, slowly arch your lower back toward the ceiling.
2. Imagine your tummy sinking towards the floor while keeping your core muscles engaged to support your lower back.
3. Lift your head and chest slightly, looking upwards (but don't strain your neck).
4. Exhale thoroughly when you reach the full arch of your spine.
5. Hold this posture for a few of breaths, feeling the stretch in your spine and chest.

Moving into Cat Pose (Inhaling):

1. As you inhale, turn your back to the ceiling like a cat.
2. Tuck your chin towards your chest without straining it. Allow the movement to emerge organically from your spine.
3. Engage your abdominal muscles and draw your navel inside, as if scooping your belly button towards your spine.
4. Concentrate on stretching your spine as you round it, experiencing a slight stretch in your back muscles.
5. Hold this posture for a few of breaths, feeling the stretch in your back and core.

Return to Table Pose:

- Exhale gently, then return to the initial table posture with a neutral spine.
- Repeat the complete sequence (from cow posture to cat pose and back) 5-10 times, or as many as you feel comfortable with.

Tips for Beginners:
1. Focus on Movement, Not Perfection: Don't obsess about having a perfectly arched or rounded back. Concentrate on the subtle movements and sensations in your spine.
2. Listen to Your Body: Move gently and attentively. If you encounter any pain, discontinue the workout and seek medical attention before resuming.
3. Breathe in as you go into cow posture (arching your back), then exhale as you move into cat pose (rounding your back).
4. Modify as needed: If kneeling is unpleasant, you can do the cat-cow stance on all fours with your hands slightly forward of your shoulders.
5. Incorporating the cat-cow position into your routine can help you achieve a more flexible and dynamic spine, better posture, and a deeper connection to your body.

Gentle Spinal Twists Pose

Spinal twists are an excellent technique to gently stretch and lengthen your spine, increase mobility, and relieve stress in your back and shoulders. As a novice, use these steps to achieve safe and effective spinal twists:

What You'll Need:

A comfortable yoga mat (optional but recommended for cushioning).

Preparation:

Find your seat: Start by sitting on the floor with your legs out in front of you. If you have tight hamstrings or find it difficult to sit with your legs straight, bend one knee and lay your foot flat on the ground.

Ground oneself by sitting tall and with a stretched spine. Imagine you're sitting bones pressing firmly into the earth for support. Relax your shoulders and lower your eyes.

The Twist:

Engage your core: Inhale deeply, then slowly shift your torso to one side as you exhale. Imagine twisting your spine, extending from your navel to your thigh.

Find your twist (avoid forcing): Do not push the twist. Go only as far as you feel comfortable and can maintain an extended spine. If necessary, place your hand on the floor behind you to provide additional support.

Breathe and hold: Keep your breathing calm and steady. Hold the twist for 5-10 relaxing breaths, concentrating on the mild stretch in your back and sides.

Engage and unwind: Inhale and slowly undo the twist before returning to center. Exhale and twist on the opposite side.

Here is some more advice for beginners:

Prioritize quality over quantity: It is preferable to focus on a mild twist with a long spine rather than forcing a deeper twist with a rounded back.

Listen to your body: If you feel any discomfort, stop twisting and return to center.

Use props for support: If sitting on the floor is unpleasant, place a bolster or folded blanket beneath your buttocks for more support.

Modify for your needs: Do not be afraid to change the twist to accommodate your body's restrictions. For example, you can maintain your upper leg bent and your foot flat on the ground, or use a chair for extra support.

Variations:

Seated Spinal Twist with Arms Up: Once you've mastered the basic twist, try raising your upper arm toward the sky for a deeper stretch in the side ribs and shoulder. Keep your lower hand on the ground behind you for support.

Supine Twist (laying Down): If seated twists are difficult, try this version laying on your back. Bring your knees up to your chest, then gradually drop one knee to the side while maintaining the other foot level on the floor. Twist your torso toward the bent knee while maintaining your shoulders firmly on the mat.

Remember:

Spinal twists are a gentle approach to increase flexibility and reduce stress. Be patient with yourself, listen to your body, and enjoy the journey of discovery!

Hips and pelvis:

Hip Circles

Hip circles are an excellent technique to warm up your hips, increase mobility, and activate your core muscles. They are a moderate yet effective workout that is appropriate for beginners of all ages and fitness levels. This is a step-by-step tutorial to guide you get started:

What You'll Need:
A pleasant location with plenty of room to roam about.
Optional: Use a strong chair or wall for increased balance.

Step 1: Stand Tall with Gentle Foot Placement.
- Start by standing tall, with your feet hip-width apart. You may alter the width slightly to achieve a more comfortable stance.
- Keep your core engaged by gradually bringing your belly button inside towards your spine.
- If you need more balancing assistance, rest your hands on a firm chair or softly touch a wall.

Step 2: Start the movement.
- Imagine that your hips are making huge circles in the air.
- Start by softly rotating your hips in a clockwise manner. Consider beginning the movement from your core and hips rather than your back.

Step 3: Concentrate on controlled movement.
- Keep the circles big and flowing, with a smooth, controlled motion.
- Avoid abrupt movements or pushing your hips beyond their comfort zone.

Step 4: Breathe deeply.

- Take deep, natural breaths while rotating your hips. Inhale as you circle ahead; exhale as you circle back.

Step 5: Complete the Set and Reverse Directions.

- Continue forming circular circles for 10-15 rounds, concentrating on feeling the movement in your hips and core.
- After you've completed your set of clockwise circles, turn directions and do 10-15 reps of counterclockwise circles.

Tips for Beginners:

- Begin with smaller circles and progressively increase your range of motion as you gain comfort and flexibility.
- **Listen to Your Body:** If you experience any pain, stop the workout and check with a healthcare practitioner before continuing.
- **Focus on Quality, Not Quantity:** It is more vital to concentrate on controlled, focused motions rather than the number of repetitions.

- **Modify for Balance:** If you require additional support, use a chair or a wall until you feel more confident.
- **Make it fun!** Put on whatever music you like and let yourself to move with your breath.

Variations:

- Once you're familiar with basic hip circles, try these variations:
- **Small Circles:** Create smaller, more controlled circles to stimulate your core more effectively.
- **Hip Isolations:** Instead of doing entire circles, focus on thrusting your hips forward, back, and side to side.
- **Raised Leg Circles:** Lift one leg slightly off the ground and make circles with your standing hip. Repeat on the opposite side.

Remember:

Consistency is crucial! Try to integrate hip circles into your routine a few times per week, even if only for a few minutes. As you grow more comfortable with the exercise, you will notice more hip mobility, better balance, and a stronger connection to your body.

Upper Body

Arm Circles

Arm circles are an excellent method to warm up your shoulders, increase upper-body mobility, and gently extend your arms. They're an excellent complement to your morning routine or for easing into a workout. Here's a step-by-step instruction for doing things safely and effectively:

<u>**What You'll Need:**</u>

Yourself and some pleasant surroundings!
Instructions:
Stand tall with proper posture: Start by placing your feet shoulder-width apart. Gently bring your belly button in towards your spine to engage your core. Maintain a lofty spine and relaxed shoulders.

Reach out to the sides: Hold your arms straight out to the sides, parallel to the ground. Imagine your arms making a large "T" with your body. Keep your elbows slightly soft and not locked.

Tiny circles, forward first: Start forming tiny circles with your arms. Imagine you're drawing little circles in the air that are approximately the size of a dinner plate. Begin by pushing your arms forward, starting with your fingers.

Concentrate on controlled movement: Move your entire arm, not just the wrists. Maintain a relaxed shoulder position and an engaged core throughout the exercise. Breathe normally throughout the rounds.

Reverse direction: After 10-15 forward rounds, smoothly reverse your direction. Imagine drawing little circles backwards, again using your fingertips to lead.

Repeat and adjust: Continue alternating forward and backward circles for 30-60 seconds (or as long as you feel comfortable). If the circles seem excessively large or create discomfort, just reduce their size.

Tips for Beginners:
- **Listen to your body:** if you observe any discomfort, stop immediately. Modify the workout as needed, for as smaller circles or shorter sets.
- **Focus on quality over quantity:** Smaller, more controlled circles are preferable to huge, choppy ones.
- progressively increase intensity: As your mobility and strength improve, you may progressively increase the size of your circles and the length of your sets.

- Make it fun! Include some amusing modifications. Make circles with your eyes closed or concentrate on feeling the stretch in different areas of your shoulders and upper back.

Arm circles can help you increase upper body mobility and connect with your body more mindfully.

Chapter 4: Release Tension in Your Hips and Pelvis: Grounding and Core Awareness

Pelvic Floor Awareness and Activation Exercises

The pelvic floor muscles act as a sling of support at the base of your pelvis. They have an important role in bladder and bowel control, sexual function, and core stability. For many women, however, these muscles can become weak or tight, causing incontinence, pelvic discomfort, and even lower back difficulties.

What is the good news? Simple exercises might help you reconnect with your pelvic floor and enhance its functionality.

Locate Your Pelvic Floor:
Before we begin the workouts, let's get to know the location. Assume you're attempting to stop the flow of pee in midstream. The muscles you need for this are your pelvic floor muscles.

Here are two mild approaches for identifying your pelvic floor:
Kegel Squeeze: While laying down, gently squeeze the muscles surrounding your urethra (where pee exits) and anus, as if raising them upward. Hold for a few seconds and then take a rest. Repeat 5 to 10 times.

Imagine the Lift: Visualize an elevator in your pelvis. As you inhale, see the elevator lowering. As you exhale, imagine it lifting up and engaging your pelvic floor muscles. Repeat a few times.

Easy Activation Exercises:

Now that you've discovered your pelvic floor, here are some exercises to activate and strengthen it:

1. Short pulses:
Lie on your back, legs bent, both feet flat on the floor.
Breathe normally. As you exhale, gently compress your
pelvic floor muscles for 1-2 seconds. Relax totally with
the inhalation.
Repeat ten times. Concentrate on quality over quantity.

2. Long Holds:
Maintain the same lying down position as before.
Inhale, and as you exhale, gently squeeze your pelvic
floor muscles for 5 seconds. Hold for the whole count,
then relax completely on the inhale.
Repeat five times.

3. Bridge:
Lie on your back, legs bent, with both feet flat on the
floor. Arms are at your sides.
Lift your hips off the ground, using your core and pelvic
floor muscles to make a straight line from your shoulders
to your knees.
Hold for 3-5 seconds and then slowly drop your hips
back down.
Repeat ten times.

Remember:

- Breathe during these workouts. Do not hold your breath!
- Concentrate on quality, not quantity. It's preferable to perform a few exercises correctly rather than many with poor technique.
- If you encounter any pain, stop exercising and get medical attention.

<u>Raising Awareness Throughout the Day:</u>

In addition to these exercises, here are some tips for incorporating pelvic floor awareness into your daily life:

- Engage your pelvic floor muscles during regular tasks, such as coughing, sneezing, or lifting something heavy.
- Maintain proper posture: Proper posture relieves strain on your pelvic floor. Stand tall, shoulders back and down.
- Stay hydrated: Drinking enough of water helps to prevent constipation, which can put stress on your pelvic floor.

By adopting these exercises and mindfulness practices, you will be able to strengthen your pelvic floor, increase your core stability, and feel better overall.

Hip Mobility Exercises to Improve Flexibility.

Tight hips may be a drag—literally! They can limit your range of motion, impede athletic performance, and possibly cause lower back pain. But don't worry, fellow explorer of mobility! Here are seven simple yet effective hip mobility exercises to increase your flexibility, all described in a beginner-friendly manner.

Remember:

- **Listen to your body:** these workouts should never cause discomfort. If you experience any discomfort, please stop and see a healthcare expert.
- Move gently and mindfully: Concentrate on the feelings in your hips and avoid jerky movements.
- Deep breathing: Inhale as you open your hips, then exhale as you release.

1. Supine Piriformis Stretch (The Butterfly Pose on Your Back):

- This exercise focuses on the piriformis muscle, which is commonly responsible for tight hips.
- Lie comfortably on your back, legs bent and feet flat on the ground.
- Gently draw your knees together, allowing them to open naturally.
- If it's comfortable, extend your arms to the sides and lay your palms on the floor.
- Hold for 30 seconds to a minute, concentrating on a slight stretch in your glutes and outer hip.

2. Figure Four Stretch:

- This stretch relaxes your outer hip and quadriceps.
- Lie on your back, knees bent.
- Cross your right ankle over your left knee, slightly above the kneecap.
- Hold your left thigh behind your knee and draw it up to your chest.
- You should feel a stretch in the right outer hip.
- Hold for like 30 seconds to 1 minute, then repeat on the opposite side.

3. Frog Squats:

- This dynamic stretch expands your inner thighs and groin.
- Stand with your feet wider than shoulder width apart, toes pointing outward.
- Squat as low as you can comfortably go while maintaining your back straight and your heels level on the floor.
- Gently push your knees outwards with your elbows to get a pleasant stretch in your inner thighs.
- Hold for 10-15 seconds before gently standing back up.
- Repeat 5 to 10 times.

4. Supine Hip Rotation:

- This workout increases your hip's internal and external rotation.
- Lie comfortably on your back, legs bent and feet flat on the ground.
- Keep your knees bent and gradually twist one leg inward, allowing your foot to land flat on the floor.
- Hold for 10 seconds, then slowly move your leg outward as far as is comfortable.

- Hold for ten seconds.
- Repeat 5–10 times on each side.

Bonus Tip:
Walking lunges with torso twists: As you lunge forward with one leg, gently twist your torso to the other direction. This introduces a rotating aspect into your hip mobility practice.

Celebrate your progress!

You may not become a contortionist overnight, but with constant practice, you will see a significant improvement in your hip flexibility. Remember: growth, not perfection, is the aim! So, keep moving, exploring, and enjoying the process of uncovering your body's possibilities.

Strengthening exercises for core stability

A strong core is necessary for proper posture, back health, and general stability. It is the powerhouse that connects your upper and lower bodies, letting you to move freely and avoid injury. But what precisely constitutes the core?

The core muscles are your abs, obliques (muscles on the sides of your waist), your back, and even your diaphragm. These exercises will target the various muscle groups, allowing you to develop core strength in a safe and effective manner.

Remember:

- Concentrate on quality over quantity. It is preferable to perform a few exercises with appropriate technique rather than many with improper form.
- Take deep breaths throughout each workout. Exhale while you engage your core, then inhale to return to the beginning posture.
- Listen to your body. If you experience any pain, stop exercising and rest.

<u>**Beginner-Friendly Core Exercises:**</u>

1. Dead Bug:
- Lay on your back, legs bent and your both feet flat on the floor. Stretch your arms straight up to the ceiling.
- Engage your core and carefully drop one arm and the opposing leg to the floor, keeping your lower back pushed against the ground.
- Try not to arching your back or lifting your hips off the floor.
- Hold for a second, then return to your starting position. Repeat for the opposite arm and leg.
- Aim for 2-3 sets of 10 reps per side.

2. Plank:
- Begin on your forearms, elbows shoulder-width apart and forearms flat on the floor. Maintain your body in a straight line from your head to heels.
- Tighten the abdominal muscles and glutes to engage your core.
- Hold this stance for as long as you can comfortably retain proper form. Start with 15-30 seconds and progressively increase the hold duration as you gain strength.

- You can start the plank on your knees rather than your forearms.

3. Bird Dogs:

- Begin on all fours, hands just beneath your shoulders, knees hip-width apart. Maintain an upright posture with a long neck.
- Engage your core and lift one arm straight out in front of you, parallel to the ground. Simultaneously, stretch the opposing leg straight back while maintaining your hip in line with your body.
- Hold for a second, then return to your starting position. Repeat for the opposite arm and leg.
- Aim for 2-3 sets of 10 reps per side.

4. Marching glute bridge:

- Lay on your back, legs bent, both feet's flat on the floor. Lift your hips off the ground and align your body in a straight line from your knees to your shoulders.
- Engage your core and glutes.
- Lift one foot off the floor and stretch your leg straight to the ceiling. Hold for a second, then return to your starting position and repeat with the opposite leg.
- Continue marching your legs for a specific period of time (30-60 seconds) or number of repetitions each leg.

Progress Tips:

As your strength increases, you can develop these workouts by:

- Increase the number of sets and repetitions.
- Holding places over a longer period of time.
- Add weights or resistance bands.
- Trying more complex variants on the exercises.

Be patient and persistent with your core workouts, and you'll eventually establish a strong and sturdy foundation for all of your activities!

Chapter 5: Awaken Your Upper Body: Shoulder and Arm Awareness

Techniques to Release Tension in the Upper Back and Shoulders.

Tension is most commonly found in the upper back and shoulders, which can be caused by poor posture, stress, or repeated activities. This tension can cause discomfort, headaches, and limited mobility. But do not be afraid! Here are some simple practices you may implement into your everyday routine to relieve stress and relax.

Gentle neck rolls:

Start Seated: Sit comfortably on a chair with your feet flat on the ground.

Slow and steady: Begin by lowering your right ear to your right shoulder, feeling a mild stretch down the side of your neck. Hold for a few breaths.

Complete the Circle: Slowly move your head forward, then up towards your left shoulder, and finally back down to the center in a circular motion. Repeat on the opposite side.

Repeat 3-5 neck rolls in each direction, with a focus on controlled movements and deep breathing.

Shoulder Shrugs (with Twist):
- **Find Your Center:** Sit or stand tall, shoulders relaxed, back straight.
- **Lift and Release:** Slowly shrug your shoulders up towards your ears, feeling the stretch in your upper back and shoulder blades. Hold your breath for a moment.
- Release and Twist: Lower your shoulders and gently roll them backward in a circular manner. Repeat 5 to 10 times.
- **Reverse it Up:** Repeat the shoulder shrugs, but this time with a forward roll. Feel the stretch in different parts of your shoulders.

Doorway Chest Opener:
Find a Doorway: Stand in a doorway, arms elevated shoulder-high against the frame's sides.
Lean In: Bend your elbows and gradually lean in from your hips until you feel a stretch across your chest and shoulders. Hold for 10–15 breaths.
Deepen the Stretch: If you feel comfortable, take little steps forward to enhance the stretch. Listen to your body and avoid putting yourself through discomfort.

Release and Repeat: Take a slow step back to the beginning posture, relaxing your arms. Repeat 2–3 times.

<u>Bonus tip: Self-Massage with a Tennis Ball!</u>

1. **Locate a Quiet Area:** Lie on your back on a mat or comfy surface.
2. **Position the Ball:** Place a tennis ball between your upper back and the wall. Lean into the ball, using mild pressure to detect any tight points.
3. **Move and Breathe:** Slowly move the ball in tiny circles, concentrating on points of tension. Breathe deeply and relax your shoulders as you let go of the strain.
4. Repeat for 30-60 seconds on each shoulder blade region. Be gentle and prevent harsh aches.

<u>Remember:</u>

- Consistency is crucial! To achieve best outcomes, use these strategies on a daily basis.
- Listen to your body. If you encounter any pain, stop exercising and get medical attention.
- Breathe deeply throughout each exercise to promote relaxation and circulation.

By implementing these exercises into your daily routine, you may successfully relieve tension in your upper back and shoulders, resulting in improved posture, range of motion, and a renewed sensation of comfort and relaxation.

Gentle stretches and mobility exercises for the arms and wrists.

Our arms and wrists are always working throughout the day, whether it's typing, carrying groceries, or reaching for the top shelf. These moderate stretches and mobility exercises can help you gain flexibility, relieve stress, and keep your arms and wrists comfortable.

<u>Remember:</u>
Breathe deeply and slowly throughout each workout.
Focus on experiencing a mild stretch rather than agony.
If you experience any pain, slow down or stop the workout.
Move gently and in control.
Wrist Circles:

Extend your arm straight in front of you, palm down.
Gently rotate your wrist in a circular motion, five times forward and five times backward.
Repeat with the opposite arm.
Finger Stretches:

<u>**Stretch one arm straight in front of you, palm up.**</u>

- With your other hand, softly draw back on your fingers to extend the top of your hand. Hold for 10–15 seconds.
- Relax your fingers and softly push down on the back of your hand to extend the palm side. Hold for 10–15 seconds.
- Repeat steps 1-3 with the opposite arm.

<u>**Prayer Stretch:**</u>

- Place your palms together in front of your chest, as if in prayer.
- Gently push your palms together and maintain your elbows relaxed. Your forearms should feel stretched. Hold for 10–15 seconds.
- Slowly stretch your elbows apart while pressing your palms together and lowering your hands to your waist. Feel the stretch go down your arms. Hold for 10–15 seconds.

<u>**Eagle Arms (Modified):**</u>

1. Extend both arms to your sides, parallel to the ground.
2. Bend your elbows and bring your forearms up to your chest.
3. Cross your right arm across your left arm, keeping your right forearm on top.

4. Gently push your palms together and elevate your elbows slightly. Your shoulders and upper back should feel stretched out. Hold for 10–15 seconds.
5. Repeat on the opposite side, crossing your left arm over your right.

Wrist Extensions:
1. Stretch one arm straight in front of you, palm down.
2. With your other hand, gently bend your wrist back and extend the top of your forearm. Hold for 10–15 seconds.
3. Relax and repeat with your other arm.

Bonus: Desk Stretch.
- If you spend a lot of time at a computer, this stretch will help reduce stress in your forearms and wrists.
- Sit at your desk with your forearms resting on the desktop and palms facing downward.
- Gently lean your upper body back, feeling the stretch in your forearms. Hold for 10–15 seconds.

Include these exercises in your everyday routine, a few times per day, or even do them while watching TV! Spending a few minutes stretching and improving mobility in your arms and wrists can keep them feeling comfortable and prepared for anything.

Exercises to Improve Upper Body Posture and Alignment

Tightness in your upper back, rounded shoulders, and a stooped posture are all frequent side effects of sitting for lengthy periods of time at a desk or using electronics. These exercises will gently stretch and strengthen your upper body muscles, resulting in improved posture and alignment.

Remember:

Breathe deeply and slowly throughout each workout.

Instead of striving for flawless form, focus on easy movements and experiencing the stretch.

Stop if you feel any pain and see a doctor if necessary.

Warm-ups (30 seconds each)

Neck Rolls: Gently roll your head in a circular motion, starting one direction and then the other.

Arm Circles: Draw little circles with your arms, first forward and then backward.

<u>**Exercises:**</u>

1. Chest Opener (focuses on tight chest muscles):
- Stand tall, feet hip-width apart.
- Clasp your hands behind your back and maintain your elbows straight.
- Gently raise your chest and push your shoulder blades together.
- Hold for 10-15 seconds and then slowly release.
- Repeat 3 to 5 times.

2. Doorway Stretch (for chest and shoulders):
- Stand in a doorway, arms outstretched high.
- Lean gently forward, keeping your arms straight and elbows near the doorframe.
- Feel a gentle stretch over the chest and shoulders.
- Hold for 10-15 seconds, then gently return to the starting position.
- Repeat 3 to 5 times.

3. Shoulder Blade Squeezes (to strengthen the upper back muscles):
- Sit or stand tall, shoulders relaxed.
- Gently push your shoulder blades together and feel them travel down your back.
- Hold for 5 seconds and then release.

- Repeat 10 to 15 times.

4. Wall Angels (enhances shoulder and spinal alignment)

- Stand with your back flat on a wall and feet hip-width apart.
- Raise your arms to the sides, elbows bent 90 degrees, forearms and palms flat against the wall.
- Slowly move your arms up the wall while maintaining your back and elbows in touch with it.
- Imagine drawing snow angels on the walls.
- Slide your arms back down the wall to the starting position.
- Repeat 5 to 10 times.

5. Row variations (to strengthen the upper back and core):

Option 1 (with resistance band):

- Stand on one leg and place your other leg slightly behind you for balance.
- Hold one resistance band in each hand, palms facing inward.
- Bend your elbows and draw the band to your chest, pushing your shoulder blades together.
- Hold for 5 seconds and then gently release.
- Repeat 10–15 times on each side.

- Option 2 (bodyweight):

Stand tall, feet hip-width apart.
- Lean slightly forward while maintaining your back straight and core engaged.
- Bend your elbows and pull your arms back as if rowing, pressing your shoulder blades together.
- Hold for 5 seconds and then gently release.
- Repeat 10 to 15 times.
- Cool-down (30 second each):

Neck Rolls: Continue the mild neck rolls from the warm-up.
Arm Circles: Perform the little arm circles from the warm-up.
Progression:

As your strength improves, you may make these exercises more challenging by holding them for longer periods of time, adding more repetitions, or using heavier weights (such as resistance bands).

Remember that consistency is crucial! For best results in improving upper body posture and alignment, perform these exercises on a daily basis.

Chapter 6: Moving Emotions: Somatic Practices for Stress Relief

The Body-Mind Connection: How Emotions Manifest Physically.

Have you ever had butterflies in your stomach before a major presentation or had a tight jaw while stressed? All of these instances demonstrate the mind-body link in action! Our emotions do not merely exist in our thoughts; they have a direct influence on our physical bodies.

Below is an explanation of how this relationship works:

The Brain and neurological System: When we feel an emotion, our brain transmits messages throughout our bodies via the neurological system.

The nervous system also causes the production of chemicals such as adrenaline and cortisol, which prepare our bodies for action (think fight-or-flight reaction).

bodily manifestations: These signals and hormones generate a variety of bodily changes, including increased heart rate, perspiration, and muscular tension.

Emotions and the Body: A Two-Way Street

It's vital to remember that the mind-body link works both ways. Emotions not only have an impact on our bodies, but our physical state may also influence them. For example, if you're tired from not getting enough sleep, you may be more irritated.

Understanding how your body communicates

Tuning into your body's signals might provide useful insights into your emotional condition. Below are a few steps to get started:

Find a Quiet Moment: Take a few moments to sit or lie down comfortably in a quiet area. Shut your eyes and minimize your gaze.

Body Scan: Imagine a gentle wave of awareness spreading through your body, beginning at your toes and gradually progressing upwards. Look for any areas of tension, tightness, or pain.

Connect the Dots: Once you've identified a bodily sense, explore what emotion could be associated with it. Does a tight chest indicate anxiety? Does a churning stomach indicate nervousness?

No judgments: There are no correct or incorrect responses here. Simply observe your body's cues without judgement.

Simple Techniques for Managing Your Body and Mind

Now that you've gained a better knowledge of this link, here are some simple techniques for managing your emotions and their physical consequences:

Deep breathing: When you're feeling stressed, take calm, deep breaths via your diaphragm. This can assist to lower your heart rate and trigger your body's relaxation response.

Progressive Muscle Relaxation: Tense and release various muscle groups throughout your body, beginning with your toes and progressing upward. This can assist to reduce bodily stress and promote relaxation.

Mindfulness Techniques: Meditation and mindful movement can help you become more aware of your thoughts and emotions in the present moment, allowing you to respond rather than react.

Physical Activity: Exercise is an excellent method to release pent-up energy and boost your mood. Select an activity that you love, such as walking, dancing, or yoga.

By being more aware of the mind-body connection, you may learn to listen to your body's cues and control your emotions in a healthy manner. Remember that caring for your physical health also benefits your mental wellness!

Somatic Breathing for Relaxation and Anxiety Relief

Have you ever noticed how your breath quickens when you're upset, or how taking a deep breath quickly makes you feel calmer? There is a strong link between your breath and your emotional state. Somatic breathwork employs this relationship to enhance relaxation and lessen anxiety.

Unlike shallow chest breathing, somatic breathwork emphasizes deep, diaphragmatic breathing. This activates your diaphragm, a big muscle beneath your lungs that allows for more full and efficient breathing. Here is how to start:

Find Your Comfort Zone:
Take a comfy pillow or blanket and lie down on your back, or sit in a chair that provides adequate back support.
Close your eyes lightly, or lessen your look if you're lying down.

Step 1: Connect with Your Breath
Position one hand on your stomach, just below the ribs, and the other on your chest.
As you slowly inhale through your nose for four counts, feel your tummy softly rise against your hand. Your chest should be reasonably motionless.

Step 2: The Power of the Pause.
After filling your tummy with air, hold your breath for a comfortable count of two.

Step 3: Release Tension

Exhale gently and thoroughly through your mouth for a count of six. Imagine blowing out a candle flame. Feel your tummy fall back down as you expel all the air.

Step 4: Repeat and observe.

For 5-10 minutes, alternate between breathing for 4, holding for 2, and exhaling for 6.

Keep an eye on your body and thoughts while you practice. Do you feel calmer? More grounded? There's no right or wrong way to feel; just observe.

Tips for Beginners:

- Focus on Comfort: If counting breaths becomes distracting, try focusing on the sensation of your tummy rising and falling.
- Listen to Your Body: Set the breath count to a rate that is comfortable for you. Do not force your breath.
- Practice Makes Perfect: As with any talent, somatic breathing requires practice. The frequent you practice, the easier it will become.

Benefits of Somatic Breathwork:

1. Decreased anxiety and stress
2. Improved relaxation and sleep
3. Improved attention and concentration
4. Improved emotional management

Beyond Relaxation:

Somatic breathwork is useful for more than simply relaxation. With practice, it may become an effective technique for dealing with challenging emotions, increasing attention, and fostering general well-being.

So, the next time you're agitated or nervous, spend a few minutes practicing somatic breathwork. You may be astonished at how quickly you may achieve inner serenity and tranquility.

Gentle movement sequences to release trapped emotions.

Our bodies store emotions. Stress, worry, and even previous injuries can cause muscular tension, chest tightness, or an overall sense of unease. Somatic movement is a gentle approach to release repressed emotions and promote calm.

Body-Mind Connection:

Consider your body to be a gigantic sponge that absorbs emotions all day. Unprocessed emotions can get trapped in certain locations, causing discomfort and tension. Somatic movement allows us to physically release pent-up sentiments, resulting in a sense of emotional and physical well-being.

Gentle movement sequences:
Here are two basic steps you may take to release imprisoned emotions:

Sequence 1: Shake It Out
This pattern relieves stress with moderate shaking motions.

- Begin standing with your feet hip-width apart and knees slightly soft.
- Let Loose: Start by lightly shaking your hands at your sides. Allow the shaking to progress up your arms and into your shoulders. Allow your body to move freely, without judgment.
- Whole-Body Wobble: Bend your knees slightly and relax your gaze. Imagine your body like a tree swinging softly in the breeze. Allow your body to move side to side, front to back, or in a circular manner.
- Ground Yourself: After a few minutes of shaking, gently stop. Take a few deep breaths and feel your feet secure on the ground.

Sequence 2: Breathe Through Tension

This practice employs concentrated breathing and mild stretches to relieve tension in the chest and belly.

- sat or Supine: Find a comfortable posture, whether sat in a chair or laying on your back.
- Deep breathing: Close your eyes and take a leisurely, deep breath in through your nose. Feel your stomach expand as you inhale. Hold for a second, then gently exhale through your lips, letting your tummy fall back down. Repeat this breath numerous times.
- Chest Opener: Inhale, extend your arms aloft and gently arch your back to open your chest. Hold for a few breaths, then gently lower your arms as you exhale. Repeat many times.
- Side Bends: Sit or stand tall, taking a deep breath in. As you exhale, gently bend your torso to one side and extend your arm above. Hold for a few breaths, then repeat on the opposite position.

<u>Remember:</u>

1. Listen to Your Body: These sequences are intended to be mild. Avoid painful motions. Modify them to match your physique and comfort level.
2. Pay attention to your breath while you move. Slow, deep breathing can assist relieve stress and promote relaxation.

3. Notice Your Emotions: As you move, take note
   of any emotions that arise. Do not try to analyze
   them; instead, notice them and let them flow
   through you with the movement.

Practice Makes Progress:
The more you practice these gentle movement patterns,
the more successful they will be at releasing stored
emotions and encouraging calm. Remember that
somatic movement is a process of self-discovery. Be
patient with yourself and appreciate the experience of
reconnecting with your body and emotions in a new
manner.

Chapter 7: Somatic practices for self-compassion and acceptance

Body-Positive Movement Practice

Somatic movement provides more than simply bodily advantages; it also serves as an effective technique for developing self-compassion and acceptance. Here, we'll look at body-positive movement methods that will help you appreciate your unique body and exercise with joy rather than punishment.

Shifting Focus:
From "Fix" to "Feel": Many traditional workout programs aim to improve your look. Body-positive movement reverses the script. Here, we concentrate on how movement feels in your body, the joy it offers, and the amazing things your body can achieve.

Let's Move with Kindness!

1. Gentle appreciation:
- Start by standing tall, with your both feets hip-width apart.
- Take a few deep breaths, allowing your tummy to rise and fall with each inhale and exhale.
- Increase your awareness of various portions of your body. Thank each portion for helping you stay strong and healthy. For example, silently thank your legs for carrying you, your arms for reaching and hugging, and your core for supporting you.

2. Loving Movement Exploration:
- Choose a moderate and gentle action, such as swinging your hips or moving your shoulders.
- Concentrate on the feelings in your body while you move. Observe any tightness or resistance, but do not force anything. Simply allow your body to move easily.

3. Celebrate your strength.
- Find a movement that feels empowering to you, such as extending your arms high or standing tall in a strong stance.
- Hold the posture for a few breaths to feel your body's power and tenacity.

4. Embrace your uniqueness:

- Move your body in a way that is joyful and enjoyable. Wiggle, shake, or dance whatever you like! There is no correct or incorrect method to move in this activity.
- Celebrate your body's unique method of expressing itself via movement.

5. Move with Gratitude:

- End your practice by laying comfortably on your back or sitting with proper posture.
- Take a few deep breaths and express thankfulness for your beautiful body.

Remember:

Body-positive movement is a journey rather than a destination. Be patient with yourself, and appreciate each step toward self-acceptance. As you walk with gentleness and gratitude, you'll develop a stronger connection and love for your unique body.

Bonus Tip: Choose a body-positive statement that speaks to you and repeat it to yourself during your practice or throughout the day. For instance, "My body is strong and capable," and "I am worthy of love and respect, just as I am."

Self-Massage Techniques for Relaxation and Tension Release.

Huh, self-massage: a lovely activity that can be performed at any time and from any location to relieve stress and promote relaxation. There is no need for sophisticated equipment; simply use your beautiful hands! These strategies are ideal for beginners and may simply be included into your regular practice.

Getting started:

- **Set the Mood:** Turn down the lights, light a candle (if desired), and play some soothing music. Make a spa-like ambiance that promotes relaxation.
- **Warm Up:** Before plunging in, spend a few minutes slowly moving your body. Roll your shoulders, extend your arms, and wiggle your toes. This prepares your muscles for massage.
- **Listen to Your Body:** Always apply light pressure while paying attention to your body's cues. If anything hurts, stop or lighten up. Self-massage should be pleasurable, not forced.

Are you ready to roll? Let's try some techniques!

1. Neck and Shoulder Release:
- Tense and Release: Sit comfortably, shoulders relaxed. Take a deep breath and tension your shoulders for a few seconds. Exhale fully, releasing all tension. Repeat a few times.
- Gently Roll: Place your fingers on one shoulder and apply gentle pressure while slowly rolling your fingers down your arm toward your bicep. Repeat on the opposite side.

2. Foot Massage:
- Roll and Release: Sit in a chair and lay a tennis ball beneath one foot. Gently move your foot back and forth over the ball, exerting pressure to any tight regions. Concentrate on the arches, heels, and toes. Switch feet and repeat.
- Squeeze and Release: Using your thumb on one side of your foot and your fingers on the other, gently squeeze your foot while moving your thumb and fingers up to your ankle. Repeat a few times and then swap feet.

3. Hand & Wrist Massage:

- Shake it Out: Begin by gently shaking your hands out, allowing your fingers to move freely. This helps relieve stress in the wrists and fingers.
- Friction Massage: Rub your palms together quickly for a few seconds to generate warmth. Then, cup one hand against the other and softly massage your palm and fingers in circular patterns. Repeat with the opposite hand.

Bonus Tip for Essential Oil Magic:

Before self-massage, use a few drops of your favorite relaxing essential oil (such as lavender or chamomile) diluted in a carrier oil (such as almond or grapeseed oil).

Remember:

Consistency is crucial! Make self-massage a regular part of your routine, even if it is only for a few minutes every day. You'll be astonished by how much stress you can relieve and how much better you'll feel.

As you grow more familiar with these techniques, you may experiment with alternative self-massage techniques that use foam rollers or massage balls to target specific muscle regions. There's an entire universe of self-care waiting to be discovered!

Cultivating Gratitude with Somatic Movement

Gratitude is a strong feeling that may elevate your spirits, increase your resilience, and deepen your connection to life. However, feeling appreciative may be tough at times, especially when things are bad. Somatic movement may be a wonderful bridge to developing a more embodied feeling of appreciation.

The body holds gratitude.
Our bodies continually communicate with us. When we are appreciative, our bodies may respond with a relaxed posture, a sigh of pleasure, or a soft smile. Somatic movement enables us to tap into and magnify pleasant bodily sensations, promoting a greater feeling of appreciation.

Here's a short, step-by-step exercise to get you started:

1. Find Your Center:

Begin by standing hip-width apart and grounding yourself. Feel the connection between your feet and the ground. Take a few deep breaths, in through your nose and out gently through your mouth.

2. Body Scan for Gratitude.

Close your eyes (optional) and focus your awareness inward. Gently check your body for any places of tension or discomfort. Exhale slowly to relieve any tightness. Now, direct your attention on places where you feel good, such as the gradual rise and fall of your chest with each breath or the warmth of the sun on your skin. Acknowledge these sensations silently and with appreciation.

3. Gentle Movement with Gratitude:

Slowly extend your arms aloft and grasp for the sky. Imagine reaching for something for which you are thankful. It might be anything—good health, wonderful relationships, or the beauty of nature. Hold this posture for a few breaths, enjoying the mild stretch in your arms and chest.

Now, slowly lower your arms to your sides, letting any tension to melt away. Imagine bringing your thankfulness down with your arms and infusing it throughout your body.

4. Expressing Gratitude via Movement:

Find a movement that seems natural to you, whether it's a gently sway, a leisurely bow, or a hand on your heart. As you travel, express your thanks, either silently or verbally. You might even say, "Thank you very much for my breath," "Thank you very much for my body," or "Thank you for [something specific you're grateful for]."

5. Integrating gratitude:

Take one last deep breath and stand tall, letting the warmth of thankfulness spread throughout your body. Carry this emotion with you throughout the day.

Remember:

- This is only the beginning point. Feel free to change the movements or add unique statements of thankfulness that speak to you.
- The goal is to be present and integrate your body and thoughts while offering thanks.
- Practice this practice on a daily basis, even if it's only for a few minutes. Over time, you'll develop a more embodied feeling of thankfulness, which will become an automatic reaction to life's benefits.

By including somatic movement into your gratitude practice, you will not only appreciate the positive aspects of your life, but also the magnificent vessel through which you may experience them - your body.

Chapter 8: Designing Your Personalized Somatic Movement Routine.

Developing a Sustainable Practice That Suits Your Lifestyle

You've started a beautiful adventure of understanding somatic movement! Now, let's develop a routine that will easily integrate into your daily life and provide long-term advantages. Here's how to create a sustained somatic practice that suits your specific lifestyle:

Step 1: Determine your "Why"
Why do you wish to add somatic movement to your routine? Is it to relieve tension, increase flexibility, or simply connect more profoundly with your body? Having a clear "why" will drive you to maintain consistency.

Step 2: Start Small and Celebrate Milestones.
Don't overburden yourself by attempting to set aside a significant amount of time each day. Start with 5-10 minutes of somatic movement. Consistency is crucial, so enjoy even minor victories!

Step 3: Find Your Best Time
Are you a night owl or an early bird? Plan your somatic practice at a time that works best for you. Perhaps it's a moderate morning ritual to wake up your body, or a relaxing sequence before bedtime to decompress.

Step 4: Make it a habit
Integrate somatic movement with your existing habits. Stretch while you wait for your coffee to make, or do some mild neck rolls while watching TV commercials. Small adjustments may make a huge difference!

Step 5: Listen to your body.
Respect your body's demands. If you're weary, go for a shorter or less strenuous practice. Remember that somatic movement is about gentle exploration rather than pushing oneself to fatigue.

Step 6: Find inspiration.
Look for tools to help keep your practice new! There are several internet videos, publications, and applications devoted to somatic movement. You can also attend local seminars or workshops to network with other practitioners.

Step 7: Embrace Variety
Explore various somatic approaches! There are other types, including Feldenkrais' gentle stretches and Body-Mind Centering's focused exercises. Find what connects with you and keeps your practice interesting.

Step 8t: Be patient and kind.
Developing a sustainable practice requires time and persistence. Do not be discouraged if you miss one or two sessions. Simply jump back in when you're ready. Be gentle to yourself and acknowledge your accomplishments along the road.

Remember:
There is no "one size fits all" solution to somatic movement. The most essential thing is to discover a practice that feels good to you and fits easily into your lifestyle. Following these steps will put you on track to gain the long-term advantages of somatic movement for your body, mind, and soul.

Integrating Somatic Movement into Daily Activities

Somatic movement is more than just devoted workout sessions. It is about maintaining a conscious connection with your body throughout the day. Here's how to easily include these activities into your everyday routine:

Tiny tweaks, big benefits.
You do not require a thorough revamp of your timetable. Begin by introducing tiny, mindful movements into your daily routine. Here's how.

Standing Up: When rising from a chair, avoid hunching. Engage your core muscles, stretch your spine, and lift yourself with your legs. Observe the change in how your body feels.

Sitting: Throughout the day, adjust your weight in your chair, roll your shoulders, and gently lengthen your neck. To avoid slouching, maintain your spine extended and shoulders relaxed.

Walking: Pay attention to how your feet feel when they make contact with the earth. Consider the natural swing of your hips and the rhythm of your breathing. Can you walk with more intention and awareness?

Climbing Stairs: Take one step at a time, concentrating on the movement of each leg and the activation of your core muscles.

Reaching: Reach for items high or low with purpose. Instead of just gripping, gently rotate your torso and feel the strain in your side.

Making It a Habit:
Set Reminders: Use your phone or a sticky note to remind yourself to engage in mindful movement throughout the day.

Begin small: Don't overload yourself. Begin with one or two activities and progressively increase as they become a habit.

Find Joy in Movement: Experiment with various forms of somatic movement, such as mild stretches, yoga positions, and tai chi. Find what feels good in your body and makes you happy.

Connect with Your Breath: Throughout the day, take several deep breaths and feel your body expand and contract. This simple act helps to focus your attention and connect with your bodily experiences.

Bonus Tip:
Transform ordinary jobs into mindful movements! While brushing your teeth, slowly extend your arms above and do side bends. Fold clothes using attentive squats or lunges. These minor alterations result in a more attentive and embodied experience in your daily life.

Remember, consistency is crucial! By implementing these modest, mindful movements into your daily routine, you will develop a stronger connection with your body and reap the numerous advantages of somatic movement throughout the day.

Find a Somatic Movement Community or Teacher (Optional)

Somatic movement may be a highly personal experience, but meeting people who share your interests can be really beneficial. While studying somatic techniques on your own is great, a community or instructor may provide significant advice, support, and encouragement. Here's a guide to help you locate the ideal match:

Step 1: Explore Online Resources:
- The International Somatic Movement Education and Therapy Association (ISMETA) provides a searchable registry of registered somatic movement educators at https://ismeta.org/. To locate practitioners near you, search by location or browse different modalities.
- Online Reviews and Recommendations: Read online reviews about local studios or somatic practitioners. Social media networks can also help you find lessons and connect with other people interested in somatic movement.

Step 2: Think about your needs and preferences.

- What do you want to learn from a community or a teacher? Are you looking for a certain modality, such as Feldenkrais or Alexander Technique? Would you prefer a drop-in class environment or a more individualized learning experience? Knowing your objectives will allow you to narrow down your search.
- What type of learning environment best fits you? Do you prefer small, intimate lessons or bigger groups? Would you prefer a compassionate and loving instructor over a more rigid approach?

Step 3: Attend a Trial Class (or Workshop).

- Many studios and practitioners provide beginning seminars or trial lessons at a discount. This is an excellent opportunity to observe various modalities and teachers firsthand. Pay attention to how you feel in class: is the lecturer clear and approachable? Does the practice appeal to your body and mind?

Step 4: Embrace the Journey

It may take some experimentation to get the ideal fit. Don't get disheartened if the first class or community isn't quite what you're searching for. Keep an open mind and enjoy the process of learning new methods to connect with your body and people who share your interest in somatic movement.

Additional Tips:

- Consult with friends, family, or healthcare professionals: They may have recommendations for local somatic movement classes or resources.
- Consider online classes: If in-person alternatives are restricted, there are several reliable online platforms that provide somatic movement classes.
- Begin small and be patient: Developing a lasting somatic movement practice requires time and effort. Begin with a moderate schedule and progressively expand your participation as you gain comfort.

Remember, the most essential thing is to locate a group or instructor that will make you feel accepted, supported, and empowered to explore the amazing world of somatic dance.

Chapter 9: Beyond the Exercises: A Journey of Self-Discovery.

The Benefits of Somatic Movement for Personal Development

Somatic movement encompasses more than just a set of exercises. It's an effective instrument for personal growth, self-discovery, and developing a stronger connection to your true self. As you move your body with intention and awareness, you'll begin on a transforming journey that goes well beyond the physical.

Introducing Body Trust and Intuition:
Traditional exercise frequently focuses on accomplishing external goals, such as weight loss or muscle building. Somatic movement teaches us to listen to our bodies and move in ways that feel pleasant. This technique cultivates faith in your body's knowledge. You'll learn to notice internal indicators such as stress, tiredness, and small changes in energy. By heeding these cues, you will have a greater faith in your body's capacity to guide you.

93

Somatic activity also increases your intuition. Paying attention to your physical sensations may reveal hidden emotions or restricting beliefs. Gentle movement and breathwork can help you eliminate emotional barriers and get access to a deeper reservoir of intuition.

Here are some strategies to tap into your body's trust and intuition.

Mindful Movement: Pay special attention to how your body feels throughout each movement while you perform somatic therapy. Observe places of tension or ease. Does a certain movement elicit an emotional response?

Body Scans: Perform body scans on a regular basis to bring your attention to different areas of your body. Feel any tightness, tingling, or warmth. This technique helps you to identify places that may require attention and release.

Set aside time for unrestricted movement exploration. Put on some music you like and let your body move spontaneously, without judgment. Allow your intuition to lead you, and watch what happens.

Embodied confidence and self-acceptance.

As you connect with your body via somatic movement, you will develop a sense of embodied confidence and self-esteem. Here's how.

Celebrating Your Body's Capabilities: Somatic movement helps you recognize your body's distinct range of motion and strength. You'll learn to move gracefully and powerfully, regardless of your size or form.

Releasing Self-Criticism: By concentrating on your body's current sensation, you may begin to let go of negative self-talk and criticism. Somatic movement encourages a more sensitive relationship with oneself.

Embracing Your Authentic Self: As you release limiting ideas and connect with your intuition, you will find your true self. Somatic movement allows you to confidently navigate through the environment and fully express yourself.

Remember:
Each woman's journey of personal growth is unique. Be patient with yourself and recognize your accomplishments, no matter how tiny. As you develop body trust, intuition, and self-acceptance, you'll experience a surge of empowerment and a stronger connection to your genuine self. Somatic movement is more than just moving your body; it is about living a more fulfilled and joyous existence.

Developing Body Trust and Intuition

As you begin your somatic movement adventure, you will learn a deep truth: your body is a source of intelligence. It conveys signals through physical sensations, guides you with subtle intuitions, and contains the secret to a stronger feeling of self-trust. In this chapter, we'll look at how to strengthen body trust and intuition, allowing you to make decisions that align with your innermost understanding.

Reclaim Your Inner Voice:
Our modern culture frequently bombards us with external signals about how our bodies should seem and act. This disconnects with our inner voice can lead to self-doubt and feelings of helplessness. Somatic movement allows us to reconnect with our inner knowledge.

Here are some strategies for developing body trust and intuition:
Tuning into Body Signals: Be aware of small bodily feelings throughout the day. Is your stomach grumbling from hunger? Do your shoulders stiffen when you are stressed? Learn to recognize these signs as important messages from your body.

The Power of "No": Allow yourself to say "no" to activities or circumstances that drain your energy or make you uncomfortable. Believe that your body's resistance is a sort of protection.

Movement as Exploration: Approach somatic movement with curiosity rather than judgment. Observe how your body reacts to various actions. Does a certain stretch feel energizing? Does another one provide a sense of grounding? Trust your body's particular inclinations.

Celebrate Non-Scale Victories: Stop obsessing about weight reduction or reaching a certain body type. Instead, focus on how your body feels: stronger, more flexible, or simply more at ease in its own flesh. Celebrate these non-scale triumphs as proof of your body's resiliency and strength.

Creating a Dialog with Your Body:

Here are a few writing topics to help you strengthen your bond with your body:

What bodily experience am I feeling right now (tiredness, warmth, tension)?

What activity feels the most nourishing to my body today?

What's one limiting idea I have about my body? How can I question it while remaining nice and compassionate to myself?

Intuition is your body's internal compass.

Your intuition is a strong instrument that communicates through gut sensations, hunches, and a sense of certainty. Somatic movement can help you become more aware of these subtle cues.

Here's how.

- **Quiet Your Mind:** Before making a choice, take a few deep breaths and concentrate on anchoring yourself in your body. Ask yourself, "How does this choice feel in my entire body?" A sensation of lightness or expansion may indicate alignment, whereas a knot in your stomach may signal the need for more thought.
- Pay attention to those unexpected "aha" moments or flashes of insight that frequently occur while movement. These might be useful guidelines for making aligned decisions.

Trusting the journey:

Cultivating body trust and intuition is a journey rather than a destination. There will be days when you feel closer to your inner knowledge than others. Accept the process with patience and self-compassion. The more you listen to your body, the more you will realize its incredible ability to direct you to a life of well-being and joy.

Remember:

You are not alone on this path. Many women have rediscovered their inner power and wisdom via somatic movement. Trust the process, respect your body's unique voice, and let your intuition lead you.

Embodied confidence and self-acceptance.

Somatic movement is more than simply physical exercises; it is a transforming path to self-acceptance and embodied confidence. As you've studied your body's sensations and actions, you've probably developed a greater understanding for its distinct strengths and skills. Now, let us build on that foundation by cultivating a sense of inner confidence.

Body Positive Movement Practices:
Celebrating Your Form: Take a few deep breaths while standing tall (or sitting comfortably). Scan your body from head to toe, recognizing each component without judgment. Take note of the shapes, lines, and posture of your body. Rather of dwelling on apparent defects, enjoy the magnificent vehicle that transports you through life.

Moving with Joy: Put on your favorite music and let your body to move naturally. There are no limits here; spin, swing, stomp, or shimmy. Celebrate the freedom of movement and the strength of your body.

Mirror Affirmations: Face a mirror and look yourself in the eyes. Repeat positive affirmations for your body and yourself. These might be simple things like "I am strong," "I am worthy," or "My body is beautiful." Say them confidently and experience the power of your own words.

Self-Massage Methods for Relaxation and Tension Relief:

Nourishing Touch: Gently massage your shoulders, neck, and scalp with your fingertips. Release any tension in these stress-related locations. As you massage, concentrate on the sensation of your touch and allow your body to melt into tranquility.

Foot pampering: Take a warm bath and treat your feet. Massage them with lotion or oil, paying special attention to the pressure spots that might help you relax all over. This simple act of self-care may be extremely calming and nourishing.

Cultivating Gratitude with Somatic Movement

Gratitude in Motion: Find a comfortable posture and take a few deep breaths. As you inhale, envision yourself feeling grateful for your body. Consider what it permits you to do: walk, dance, and embrace loved ones. Exhale and let go of any negative thoughts or self-doubts.

Moving with Intention: Incorporate tiny acts of appreciation into your daily routine. Stretch your arms upwards while silently thanking your body for its power. Take a deep breath and appreciate your lungs for providing you with life. Integrating gratitude into your somatic practice promotes a stronger connection and respect for your body.

Remember:
Embodied confidence and self-acceptance are journeys rather than destinations. There will be days when negative ideas emerge. The goal is to be patient with yourself and regularly apply these approaches. As you cultivate a healthy relationship with your body, you will

naturally exude radiant confidence that stems from inside.

Accept the real you. Your body is a powerful and wonderful vehicle deserving of love and respect. Move with delight, embrace your form, and let your inner confidence show!

Conclusion

Congratulations! You've gone on an incredible adventure of self-discovery through somatic movements. You've probably seen a difference as you've experimented with moderate workouts, increased your body awareness, and welcomed your senses. Perhaps you move more freely, breathe deeply, or get a new respect for your body.

This, my dear reader, is the transformational impact of somatic movement on women. It's more than simply exercise; it's a journey to reclaim your body and mind.

A journey of reintegration
Somatic movement has helped you close the gap between your mind and body. You've learnt to listen to your body's murmurs rather than its yells. This increased understanding enables you to make decisions that are beneficial to your well-being, cultivating a sense of self-compassion and acceptance.

Beyond The Physical:
The benefits go well beyond the physical. Somatic movement promotes emotional health and resilience by releasing imprisoned emotions and promoting self-compassion. It enables you to tap into your inner power and face life's obstacles with more confidence.

A Lifelong Practice:
Remember that somatic movement is a lifetime practice, not a goal. There will be days when mild movement seems like the right medication, and others when silence is the greatest option. Accept the journey, try new methods, and see what resonates with you.

Finally, embrace your authentic self.
As you continue your investigation, keep in mind that there is no one-size-fits-all method. This practice focuses on appreciating and embracing your individual body's requirements. You deserve to move in a way that feels nice as well as looks beautiful.

Somatic movement enables you to release cultural expectations and accept your true self. Move with joy, purpose, and the conviction that you are capable of living confidently and lovingly in your body.

May your path remain one of self-discovery, empowerment, and connection.